Walking Kung

Walking Kung

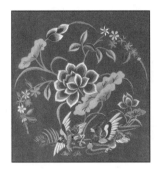

BREATHING FOR HEALTH

Sheng Keng Yun

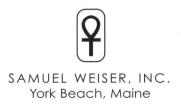

SAMUEL WEISER, INC.
York Beach, Maine

First published in 1997 by
SAMUEL WEISER, INC.
Box 612
York Beach, ME 03910-0612

Library of Congress Cataloging-in-Publication Data

Sheng, Keng Yun.
    Walking Kung : breathing for health / Sheng Keng Yun.
        p.   cm.
    Includes index.
    ISBN 0-87728-895-X (pbk. : alk. paper)
        1. Ch'i kung. 2. Breathing exercises. 3. Fitness walking.
    I. Title.
    RA781.8.S535   1997
    613.7'1--dc21   97-1467
                                                                 CIP

ISBN 0-87728-895-X
MG
Typeset in 11.5 Truesdell
Cover and text design by Kathryn Sky-Peck

Printed in the United States of America

03 02 01 00 99 98 97
10 9 8 7 6 5 4 3 2 1

The paper used in this publication meets the minimum requirements of the
American National Standard for Permanence of Paper for
Printed Library Materials Z39.48-1984.

Contents

Part 1:
Introduction to Chi Kung

Part 2:
Walking Kung

THIS BOOK IS DEDICATED to the memory of my father and mother. My father, a Taoist, inspired me to study Ch'i Kung and Tai Chi Chuan. From the time I was 5 or 6 years old, he would take me to watch demonstrations of every kind of Ch'i Kung, martial arts, Tai Chi Chuan. These left a deep impression in my mind. My mother, a devout Buddhist, worshipped regularly, and I went with her many times to the temples. This also left a deep and lasting impression on me. Both parents taught me to be kind, to help others in any way I could, and to do beneficial things for my fellow human beings.

Foreword

 SINCE I HAVE had forty-five years of exploring and studying Asian history and the arts of Asia I thought there was little from that part of the world that I had not at least heard of. As a result, it came as quite a surprise to me when I first heard Professor Sheng Keng-Yun speak of Ch'i Kung. Just why this ancient Chinese form of exercise and medicine should have remained a carefully guarded Chinese secret for so long, and why it is still largely unknown in the West, continues to be a mystery, but I am personally delighted that our ignorance of Ch'i Kung is about to come to an end.

Of course Professor Sheng's contribution is much greater than merely having written about Ch'i Kung. She has also been teaching large numbers of enthusiastic Americans to practice Ch'i Kung and to directly receive the benefits of its healing powers.

Now she has produced a basic book, one which explains both the underlying philosophy as well as the techniques of Ch'i Kung. In a very short time, Professor Sheng has done much to make Ch'i Kung accessible to Americans.

I only hope this will not be her last English language text on the subject. I hope she will now produce other books which will introduce the American people to more advanced levels of Ch'i Kung.

Those of us who have had the pleasure of knowing Professor Sheng personally know how enthusiastic she is, and how dedicated she is to converting everyone she meets to the practice of her art. This book will surely carry her a long way toward achieving that goal.

Robert Kohls, Ph.D.
Director, Office of International
Programs
San Francisco State University

Acknowledgments

I AM GRATEFUL to Professor Robert Kohls; to Judith Faria; to her daughter, Nicole Piscionere; to Robert Lew and Gary Dulberg; and to my friends and all my students for their generous help with the preparation of my book.

Publisher's Note

THE AUTHOR and publisher of this material are not responsible in any manner whatsoever for any injury caused directly or indirectly by reading or following the instructions in this text. The physical and psychological activities described in the text may be too strenuous for some people. Readers of this text should consult a qualified physician before engaging in these, or any other, exercises.

If you have a medical condition, or are of uncertain health, immediately seek attention and advice from a qualified medical doctor. Although the practice of Chi Kung is beneficial in many instances, it is neither a diagnostic tool nor an exclusive treatment for pathological conditions. Chi Kung can be used to complement, but not replace, a doctor's care.

Chi Kung—Vital Energy for Life

It is the law of Nature
Which people have always believed;
That human beings made of earth
Are connected with the heavens.

Chi Kung—vital energy for life
It will nourish you
And prolong your life.

It is very precious
To cultivate virtue all your life
No matter
What you do, or
Where you are.

To practice relaxation, to be tranquil,
To be in a natural state—
These are the hallmarks of Chi Kung.

A powerful consciousness of vital energy
Will radiate from your heart;
From this energy flows
A wonderful spirit of peace and love
From you to others,
To nature and to the cosmos.

We will all improve ourselves
By learning Chi Kung—the vital energy for life.

Preface

WHEN I WAS very little, still a baby, my mother liked to dress me in little boy's clothing. Why did my mother like to dress me like a boy? I was told afterward that it was because she had given birth to three girls, including me. She was longing to have a little boy, so she dressed me in a boy's hat, shoes, and clothes. I became used to it. At that time, I may have even thought I was a boy, so, when I was about 4 or 5 years old, I played with boys rather than with girls. One day I followed the boys to climb tall trees in order to look for eggs in birds' nests. I fell from the tree, but although my arms and back were very painful, I did not cry, but acted very bravely. When I returned home, I did not tell my parents. Sometimes I followed those boys to the suburbs to catch crickets. I found a cricket and brought it home. I carefully fed it with tender green grass. Sometimes I brought it to fight with the boys' crickets. Mine would always win and this made me very happy.

I was a very active and curious child, asking many questions. My father invited a private tutor to come to our house to teach me to read and write the ancient Chinese classical language.

I also studied in the Kwen Hua Girls Middle School, in Kunming, Yunnan Province, in southwest China. This is a very famous school. I was there for six years. While I studied there, I also pursued gymnastics, volleyball, and basketball in addition to maintaining a high average. Under the president, there were three directors: one was responsible for teaching, one for training moral character, and one for gymnastics and sports. The school regulations were very strict. Every student had to abide by the rules or be expelled. Students wore uniforms. In spring and summer, the uniforms had white, short-sleeved shirts with blue silk embroidery, black skirts, and white shoes and stockings. In autumn and winter, the uniform was the same except the shirts

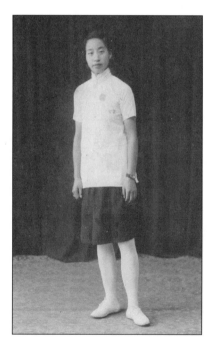

were blue and had long sleeves embroidered with the name of the school in white silk.

In 1949, I graduated from Yunnan University with a degree in foreign languages and literature. Because of China's close relations with the Soviet Union at the time, there was a high demand for Russian language speakers in China. Since there were no Russian language courses available at my university, I was sent to the Institute of Foreign Languages at Harbin in northeast China, where I studied Russian for two years. Returning to Yunnan University, I began teaching Russian, and because there was great interest in learning the language, I quickly became overloaded with course work, teaching four classes at three levels on a regular basis. Naturally, the pace at which I worked placed me under constant pressure and the increasing stress allowed me no time for relaxation.

In 1955, I became very ill, suffering from rheumatism, neurasthenia, and hypertension, which caused me to be hospitalized. The combined symptoms of these illnesses made it impossible for me to speak in anything more than a weak low voice. I was unable to walk, or even sit up in my bed, and I could not sleep for many days at a time. Realizing that neither Western medicine nor traditional Chinese medicine would be able to cure me, my family took me out of the hospital and brought me home.

This was the first time in my life that I had been seriously ill. I had always been very healthy and athletic. Now I was help-

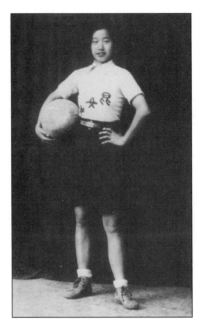

less, unable to move, and I was frightened. The doctors couldn't seem to find a cure for my condition and had told my parents that I would die.

Hoping to save my life, my father invited a famous Chi Kung master to our house to instruct me in Chi Kung. I remember being excited at the prospect of meeting this master and I can vividly recall our first encounter: "If you believe in Chi Kung, you will be healed," he said, "but if you do not believe, then I can do nothing." I could only nod my head to show that I believed.

At first it was almost impossible for me to practice Chi Kung. I could not stop worrying about dying. I was unable to quiet my mind, and even the simplest movements were quite difficult. Gradually, however, under the direction of the master, I learned to concentrate. Slowly I was able to sit up, could sleep at night, and was able to walk across my room. After one year of this practice my condition had greatly improved and I decided to learn more about Chi Kung.

Shortly after this, I was informed that a Tibetan Buddhist Chi Kung Master and poet, Lin Gar Den Ba, was visiting Huating Temple at Dian Chi Lake near Kunming. My friend, Chen Yion Chin, and I decided that we would go to the temple together to meet him. Lin Gar Den Ba was about 90 years old at the time, but his face was the rose-pink color of a baby's skin, and when we saw him, we immediately felt peaceful and relaxed. Without speaking, he gestured for us to sit down with him. Then he poured us each a cup of fresh spring water and began to write this poem with his brush:

> *With your friend, Chen Yion Chin,*
> *You visit me on the Western Mountain.*
> *Your spirit is heavy with illness.*
> *Lightness and Tranquillity come with courage.*
> *One cup of clear spring water*
> *will wash away your worries.*
> *Originally, you had no sickness*
> *yet now you knit your brow!*

Obviously, Lin Gar Den Ba recognized that I was not completely well.

We spent several days at the temple and slept in a room directly below the master's quarters. I still had discomfort in my back, and I suffered from persistent fears. I told the master about these things and he encouraged me to be brave. The first night my fears became an overwhelming burden to me, and I cried out loudly in the dark. Suddenly, to my surprise, I heard the master's powerful voice call out to me from his room, "Don't cry," he said, "Turn onto your right side. Straighten your right leg. Bend your left leg on top of it. Place your right hand on the pillow with your palm touching and holding your cheek, and rest your left hand comfortably on your left thigh." Following these instructions I was able to sleep soundly for the remainder of the night.

The next day, this great master taught me the "Conquer the Devil Kung" in order to help me drive away my fears. He instructed me to recite the Buddhist charm "On, Ah, Hon" and then to shout loudly the word "Pei!" while heavily stamping my foot on the ground. Although this may sound silly to you, it really helped me overcome my fears, and I continued to practice this Kung whenever I was afraid. Eventually, my fears disappeared for good. Before leaving the temple we joined the more than one hundred monks who had gathered there to pray and chant, and shared a delicious vegetarian banquet that I fondly remember to this day.

My friend, Chen Yion Chin, and I were to meet Lin Gar Den Ba again when he was invited to teach Chi Kung to the patients at Kan Fu Hospital near our homes in Kunming.

During this time of study, the master taught us a quiet form of Chi Kung called "Natural Meditation." When the weather was good, he would take us for walks and we would each carry a small wooden stool until we reached some beautiful spot, where we would stop and sit for an hour. He told us to keep our eyes open and ourselves receptive to our surroundings so that we could quietly absorb the sights and the fresh air of nature. When we returned to the hospital, we would meditate with our eyes closed and recall all the beauty and peace of our walk. Lin Gar Den Ba then told us to let the beautiful scenery live in our minds so as to make us happy and comfortable, relaxed and peaceful. We also learned several other sets of Chi Kung from him, including the "Eight Lotus Petal Kung" which is very helpful in improving the kidneys.

One year after I had met this man, I completely recovered from the ailments that once threatened to take my life. My whole life had changed thanks to the miraculous heritage of Chi Kung, and I decided to devote my time to study this priceless gift to humanity. I traveled to Suchou, Beijing, Hangchou, Shanghai, and Nanjing, studying with many famous masters from whom I learned more than thirty sets of Chi Kung and Tai Chi Chuan. Then I returned to Kunming, took up my foreign languages teaching duties at Yunnan University, and continued to practice and research Chi Kung in my spare time.

In 1985, I came to the United States. In 1989, I received a certificate for completing the Special Training Program of the

Exchange Scholars Program at San Francisco State University. There I studied Traditional Chinese Medicine, English Creative Writing, and Russian. Meanwhile, I taught Chi Kung there for five years. In October of 1993, I received Permanent Resident Status in the United States.

In China I was invited to join the Chinese Chi Kung Scientific Academy. Membership was offered only after the academy received many testimonial statements from students to prove that, after they practiced the Chi Kung taught by me, they recovered from their individual diseases.

For more than 40 years, I have been learning, researching, practicing, and teaching many forms of Taoist, Buddhist, and Medical Chi Kung, as well as various forms of Tai Chi Chuan. I have gained so much from the many great masters who have enriched my life with their knowledge that I would like to contribute what I have learned to others who might be interested in this art form to improve and maintain their health. I do hope that the people who read this book will practice the techniques and use these systems to heal themselves.

PART 1

Introduction to Chi Kung

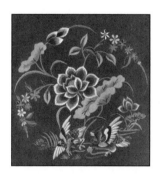

*Practicing Chi Kung for one day,
One will receive a day's benefit.
If one stops practicing [Chi] Kung for one day,
It will be equivalent to losing one hundred days' benefits.
If one stops practicing for one hundred days,
One will get no benefit through all his or her life.
Life will become an empty dream.*

—ANCIENT CHINESE PROVERB

General Principles of
Practicing Chi Kung

 IN CHINA, there are many different styles of Chi Kung. In ancient China, there was no Chi Kung school or college. Until recent times, the masters only taught their disciples during private lessons. This book explains only one style.

Before you work with the exercises, you should know what Chi Kung means. Literally, Chi means "air" or "breath"; it is pronounced "Chee." Kung means "working of," and is pronounced "Goong." In the Pinyin system of Chinese writing, you would call Chi Kung "Qigong," but in this book I have chosen what is easier for Americans to pronounce, since many people in the West are more familiar with the older Wade Giles system of translating Chinese.

Chi refers to the vital energy present in all living things. Thus, Chi Kung literally means "the working of air or breath," but it is more complicated than this, because it refers to the working of the invisible vital energy in the human body. Chi is the vital energy which animates all organisms; you cannot live without Chi. It is found wherever there is life: from the moment of conception to the moment just before death, Chi is present, being consumed and constantly being replenished. It is present wherever there is movement. Chi is the source of growth and vigor in all living things, including plants, animals, and micro-organisms. There is no exact equivalent to the concept of Chi in Western science, but Chinese scientists regard Chi as a substantial material that has been objectively verified to exist. Chi Kung is the internal function of conscious thought which is the highest stage of activity in the cerebral cortex.

What is Kung? "Kung" means the time and quality of the practice of working with Chi. Kung also describes the process of learning the methodology and the attainment of the skill necessary for successfully practicing Chi Kung. In short, Kung is the method by which you can build up Chi. Through Chi Kung practice, true Chi is made to function normally and exuberantly inside the human body. The Chinese people know that the practice of Chi Kung can cure many kinds of diseases. There are many methods and techniques that can be used to heal sickness, and the effects of various techniques or "styles" are different. If a patient goes to a hospital, she may receive X-rays, injections, acupuncture or medicinal herbs. This is a passive form of treatment, and is used by allopathic doctors.

Practicing Chi Kung is an active form of treatment. Why? It is because practicing Chi Kung can increase one's life force and immunity to diseases. As the patient practices Chi Kung, the body will become more healthy and stronger than before.

Gradually one is able to use one's own internal Chi to adjust the Yin and Yang within the body to dredge one's meridian pathway.

The Chi will flow to every part of the body, thus eliminating the illness. According to the theory of Chinese medicine: Where there is pain, there, the Chi cannot pass through. Where there is no pain, there Chi can pass through fluently. The body will eventually become more flexible than before. This is the way in which one can use internal Chi to cure one's own sickness. That is why this method is an active form of treatment.

Before you practice Chi Kung, it is necessary to develop confidence, determination, and perseverance. All three are very important. Before you start to practice Chi Kung, you should have firm confidence, ambition, determination and steadfastness. Perseverance, above all, is the most important.

First of all, you must believe in Chi Kung before you can diligently and seriously practice it. The effect will be evident and great. Here is a Chinese proverb: "Catch fish for three days, but expose the net in the sun for two days." The effect will not be good enough. Diligent and serious practice of Chi Kung is the first important condition.

Next is determination. When you believe that Chi Kung can heal your chronic diseases, you should be determined to practice very diligently. Day by day, the effect will get better. You know and feel that the energy has increased more than before. In this way, the determination becomes more firm and ambitious.

The third condition is perseverance. You must practice Chi Kung every day. Do not care if the weather is fine or rainy. You should be unwavering in practicing Chi Kung. Constantly practicing will increase your life force and immunity to disease. It will also return your youth and enable you to obtain longevity.

Great numbers of people are practicing the ancient Chinese Walking Kung to increase the life force and immunity to disease in China today. This practice makes the body healthy. It helps make you mentally and physically stronger and healthier, and even helps to fight against such modern diseases as the much-feared cancer. The effect is great and powerful. Do not hurry; practice gradually, according to your body's condition—not beyond. Each time you practice, you should feel comfortable. Do not practice so much that you become exhausted.

Functions and Effects of Walking Kung

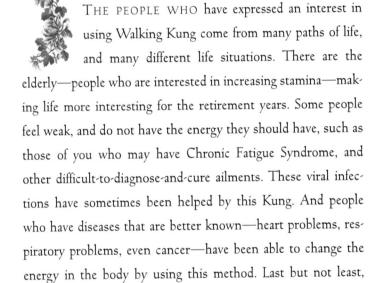THE PEOPLE WHO have expressed an interest in using Walking Kung come from many paths of life, and many different life situations. There are the elderly—people who are interested in increasing stamina—making life more interesting for the retirement years. Some people feel weak, and do not have the energy they should have, such as those of you who may have Chronic Fatigue Syndrome, and other difficult-to-diagnose-and-cure ailments. These viral infections have sometimes been helped by this Kung. And people who have diseases that are better known—heart problems, respiratory problems, even cancer—have been able to change the energy in the body by using this method. Last but not least, there are healthy people who want to encourage the immune system, reduce stress, keep the body fit in this busy world, and this group will also benefit from Walking Kung.

An ancient Chinese proverb says, "When the Chi (life force) is flowing fluently throughout every part of my body, how can disease attack me?"

Older people, or those who find their physiological functions decreasing day by day, realize that the body is sometimes
unable to renew its physiological functions as it did in youth or
in health. Walking Kung produces special benefits for these people. Walking Kung may even help cure some chronic diseases, by
improving the digestive system, the immune system, the respiratory system, the nervous system. It helps soften and relax the
joints and makes the body more flexible. All of this can be
accomplished without exerting any strength, which is what
makes this Kung so beneficial. This is an easy Kung to learn.

As you walk, you must let the following phrases pass
through your mind:

> *Mind thinking nothing;*
> *Body relaxed and tranquil;*
> *Inhaling more oxygen than exhaling!*

If your mind is quiet and peaceful, and empty of thoughts as you
practice, your physical and mental strength will increase consid-
erably, and your blood circulation will flow in a healthy manner.
Gradually, you will begin to notice that your chronic diseases are
getting better, and you will be on your way to recovery.

Athletic activities of various kinds can benefit many people, but not every kind of sport is of benefit to older or weak
people. Take running, for example. It can improve the muscles
and it can improve the blood circulation. But, if the muscles are

in great tension, the blood circulation condition could become worse. On the contrary, when the muscles are relaxed, the blood circulation inside the muscle will increase. From this point of view, it is better not to use body strength. When the mind thinks nothing and relaxes, the blood circulation will increase many times more than when you use strength on the body and put the mind into a state of great tension.

Chi Kung Breathing

THE ANCIENT CHINESE KUNG is essentially a basic breathing and walking exercise.

There are 17 kinds of breathing methods. Usually, inhaling and exhaling is considered as one breath. The length of the breath in these methods is not the same, you can inhale and exhale only once for three minutes, or you can inhale and exhale three times in one minute. In another exercise called "Tortoise Breathing Kung," inhalation can last a long time. First, I will mention 9 kinds of breathing Kung:

1. Natural Respiration

This is an instinctive physiological phenomenon which is not necessarily controlled by your consciousness. The breathing movement is natural, soft, and smooth, but rather superficial. Inhale and exhale with the nose.

2. Favorable Breathing

As you inhale, your abdominal wall will protrude or convex, so that the diaphragm is descended. When you exhale, the abdominal wall becomes concave and the diaphragm is ascended. It should be used to achieve a greater amplitude of diaphragmatic and abdominal wall movement. This type of abdominal-wall-breathing is effective for the treatment and prevention of cardio-vascular and cerebro-vascular diseases.

3. Reverse Respiration

The movements of the diaphragm and abdominal wall are just the reverse of favorable respiration. The amplitude and strength of movement are also greater than the favorable type, because, as you inhale, your abdominal wall becomes more concave, and the diaphragm will be ascended. During exhalation, your abdominal wall will become convex, and the diaphragm is descended.

4. Holding Respiration

There are two types, one of which is to consciously prolong the time of expiration, while the other prolongs the inspiratory dura-tion. Holding and Reverse Breathing are often used to treat and prevent digestive diseases.

5. Nasal Inhale and Oral Exhale

This type of breathing is applied to patients whose nasal or res-piratory passage is constricted and too narrow. Normal respira-tion is to inhale and exhale with the nose. It is better for the res-piratory system.

6. Ventilation Through the Du and Ren Channels

This method is good for the prevention and treatment of nervous diseases. The practitioner adopts reverse breathing to inhale with the nose. At the same time, he or she must imagine that the Chi (vital energy) is directed to the Dan Tian (three fingers below the navel) and then to the perineum region. After that, he or she must imagine that the Chi is passing from the perineum region up through the spinal column to the top of the head (the Bai Hui or crown of the head) to be exhaled through the nose. This is termed the "lesser respiratory cycle" of breathing.

7. Squatting and Standing Respiration

As you squat, slowly embrace the front of your knees with both hands, palms inward and exhale. Inhale as you stand up slowly. See figures 1 and 2.

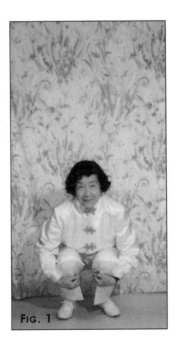
FIG. 1

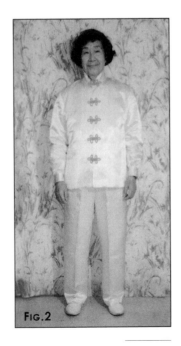
FIG. 2

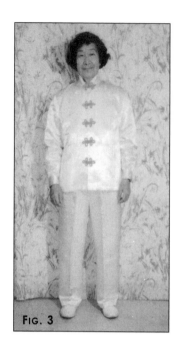
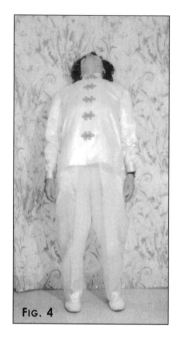

FIG. 3   FIG. 4

8. Stretch to Inhale, Erect to Exhale

Stand quietly with feet parallel and as wide as your shoulders. Then, stretch your torso, head and upper part of the body backward and inhale. Return your body to an erect standing position and exhale. See figures 3 and 4.

9. Rough Breathing

When you inhale and exhale, you can hear your breathing sound: a "shi shi" sound with each inhale and a "hu" sound with each exhale. See Five-Step Walking Kung on page 81.

It is advisable to choose a breathing method suitable for your condition. However, you should change your respiration into a normal type after 5, 10, or 15 minutes of exercise, no matter which method you select. Your muscles will become over-strained and results could be dangerous to the body if you do not. An old saying used to describe the latter condition as "tangled by the ghost to go too far."

You must pay attention to the combination of practice and rest; that is, the practice of breathing should be connected with resting. Practice for a while, then rest for a while. In this way, you will achieve a natural, smooth, and gentle breathing under the direction of fundamental principles. You should not be over-anxious for quick results. Go step-by-step slowly to achieve deep, smooth, and gentle breathing. Never hurry!

The lung capacity differs among people. Some people have a large capacity, and some have a small capacity. The former can inhale much more oxygen and fresh air. Age or gender makes no difference. From your lung capacity, we may know something about your health. For example, if one person is 20 years old, and another is 40 years old, and the lung capacity is the same, the health condition of both is about the same. If a person has a large lung capacity, he or she can inhale a lot of oxygen and fresh air, which can improve health, blood circulation, etc.

How can you inhale more oxygen? The trees emit a lot of oxygen and absorb carbon dioxide in the evening. Wherever there are trees, you should go there to practice Chi Kung so that you can absorb oxygen. Eventually, very slowly, it will enlarge your lung capacity. If you go to the forest or the park, it is best to go early in the morning so you can exchange respiration with the trees. The trees inhale your carbon dioxide, and you inhale their oxygen. You and the trees take what you need from each other.

Remember to pay attention to the two training methods: one is to train your breathing; the other is to train your walking.

Chi Kung Breathing and Walking

ASCENDING AND DESCENDING; opening and closing: these are terms you will encounter in the study of Chi Kung. We will now define several different types of breathing patterns and exercises that you will use in Walking Kung.

Dan Tian Three-Breathing

The method of Dan Tian Three-Breathing is to continuously inhale and exhale by inhaling through the nose and exhaling through the mouth. This is the best way to let the mind gradually become quiet and to be completely at rest.

• Beginning posture

Stand naturally with your feet shoulder width apart and hands down by your sides as shown in figure 5 on page 18. Before starting to breathe, relax your whole body. Don't force yourself to exhale or inhale. Just practice breathing naturally. One inhale, combined with one exhale, is called "one breath."

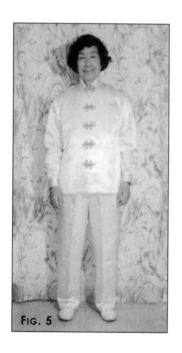

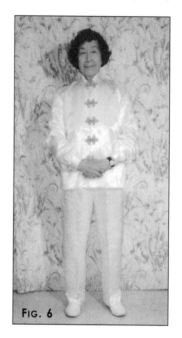

Fig. 5   FIG. 6

1. Move your hands slowly together from the sides of the thighs to the Dan Tian (the Dan Tian is located three fingers width below your navel). Both palms are opposite each other. Slowly move them up toward the abdomen; then turn the palms to the inside, facing the body. Cross your hands with the Inside Laogong (see glossary) of the right hand against the Outside Laogong of the left hand. See figure 6.

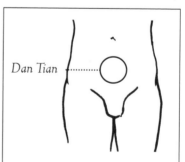

Dan Tian

Called the "sea" for the Chi of the whole body; used as a consciousness point and to store Chi energy.

2. Start to breathe. First exhale through the mouth, then inhale with the nose. This is done to replenish the weak body. During breathing, relax your waist and thighs. Breathing is natural; don't force yourself to breathe deeper or longer. Natural breathing does not use conscious thought to conduct the movement of Chi. Practice three times.

The Inside Laogong and Outside Laogong points are very important acupuncture points. Inside Laogong is in the palm of your hand; Outside Laogong is on the back of your hand, exactly opposite your Inside Laogong (see illustration below). These points stimulate the function of the heart and protect the kidneys. They can help cure heart disease, hypertension, inflammation of the joints, and high or low fevers. In China these points are used to prevent and heal various chronic diseases or cancer.

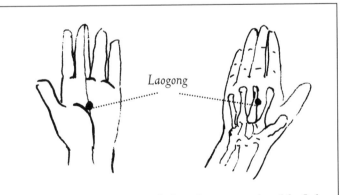

Inside Laogong is the point inside the palm at inner edge of the fleshy part of the thumb. The Outside Laogong is exactly opposite this point on the back of your hand.

Dan Tian Three Opening and Three Closing

When you have finished Three-Breathing, slowly separate your hands. Hold your hands with the backs together, palms outward, and the fingers closed naturally. Move your hands apart to shoulder width, or a little wider, keeping the elbows bent. This movement is called "One Opening." See figure 7.

After Opening, turn both hands slowly so that the centers of the palms face each other. Move them together in front of the abdomen toward the Dan Tian until both hands almost touch. This movement is called "One Closing." Repeat Opening and Closing 3 times. This part requires that the Inside Laogong and

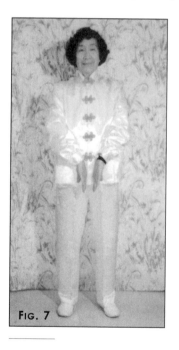

FIG. 7

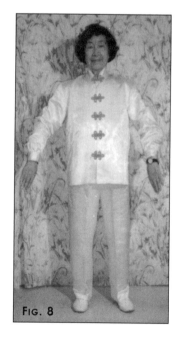

FIG. 8

Outside Laogong of both hands are opposite each other in order to stimulate the function of the heart and protect the kidneys. Gradually, you will begin to feel the Chi flowing between your hands and centering in the Dan Tian (three fingers width below the navel.) See figure 8.

Ascending and Descending, Opening and Closing

1. Do the Beginning Posture (page 17).

2. Move your left leg and foot forward and shift the weight of your body to the right leg and foot. Then slightly lift the left foot off the ground, step forward and let the heel touch the ground first with the toes up. Then let the toes fall down slowly.

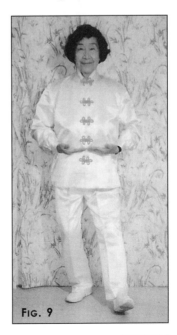

3. Move both hands slowly together from the left and right side toward the Dan Tian, palms upward and flat, with the long fingers of the hands almost touching but not actually touching, as shown in figure 9.

FIG. 9

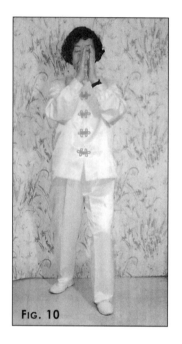

FIG. 10

4. Ascending Style. To do this posture, move your hands up slowly along the abdomen and chest. Continue up over the head. While ascending, relax your shoulders, allowing elbows and wrists to sink. Use your hands to lead the arms up (figure 10). The front foot does not move while the gravity of the body slowly moves forward. When the front foot is put flat, the heel of the back foot natu-rally lifts up and the toes remain in the same place. The body does not bend forward, the shoulders should not lift up, nor the waist contract.

5. Then change the position of your hands. Turn your fingers, pointing upward, so that the centers of the palms are facing inward. Raise the hands to

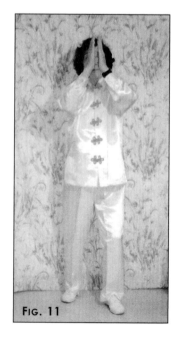

FIG. 11

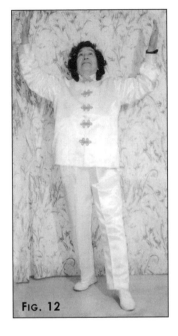

FIG. 12

Yingtan, the point above and between the eyebrows (see figure 11).

6. Opening Movement. This position requires that you move your hands as wide as the shoulders or a little wider. The back of your hands should face each other. Hold this position. During the Opening, the gravity of the body gradually moves from the front leg to the back leg. Balance the body on the right back foot, and lift the toes of the left foot slightly. The front (left) foot holds no weight. The upper part of the body slightly bends back. See figure 12.

7. When finishing Opening, slowly turn your wrists so that the centers of the palms are opposite each other.

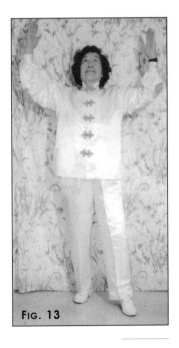

FIG. 13

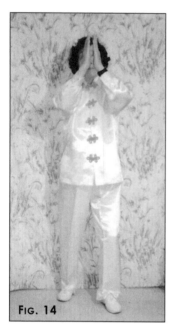

FIG. 14

Hold this position for a little while. See figure 13.

8. Ascending Closing Style. Move both hands slowly to Yingtan, almost touching hands, gradually moving the gravity of the body from the back leg to the front leg. The heel naturally lifts up a little bit. See figure 14.

9. Descending Style. When both hands have closed in front of the Yingtan, turn the tips of the extended fingers toward each other, palms flat and facing downward. Bring hands down from Yingtan to Dan Tian. See figure 15.

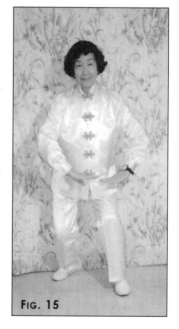

FIG. 15

10. While both hands descend, slowly let the body sink until you have reached a squatting position. Flatten the front foot with the back leg bending to squat and the toes touching the ground. When squatting, it is very necessary to do so very slowly. Try to keep the upper part of the body stable, and relax the waist until the hands descend in front of the knees. Do not force yourself to squat too low. Practice squatting as far as you can naturally. See figure 15.

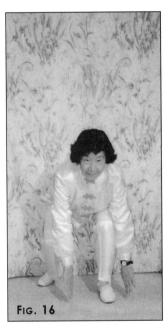

FIG. 16

11. Descending Opening Style. With the hands pressing down from the squatting position, at the same level as the knees, rotate the wrists so that your fingers point downward and the backs of the hands face each other, palms facing outward. See figure 16.

12. Open the hands as wide as the shoulders. Rest a while, relax the shoulders and elbows, and let the wrists hang loosely.

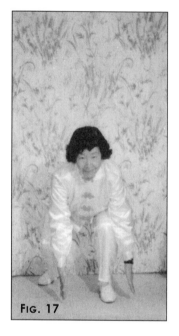

FIG. 17

13. When finishing Opening, slowly rotate the wrists so that the palms face each other with the tips of the fingers slanting outward and downward. See figure 17.

14. Then, slowly, move to the Closing position in front of your knees, moving your hands from the outside to the inside. Stay in the squatting position. With conscious thought, let the hands hang.

15. Raise your hands, palms still facing each other, to the middle of your chest. Meanwhile, move the waist and bring your legs slowly back to the standing position. The weight of your body should move back to the back right foot, and the

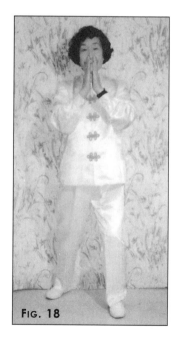

FIG. 18

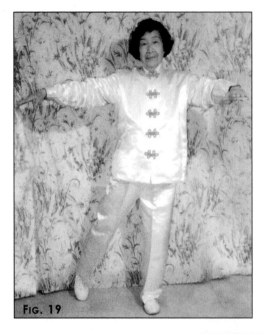

FIG. 19

back foot be-
comes flat. See
figure 18.

16. Turn palms
downward and
in front of Dan
Tian. See figure
19. Separate the
hands and arms
and let them
hang naturally
by the sides of the body. At the
same time, draw back the right
leg to the starting position. The
gravity of the body is now
falling between both legs. At
the end, the hands are brought
together in front of the Dan
Tian. That means that you are
collecting your Chi in your Dan
Tian. Figure 20 shows the starting position.

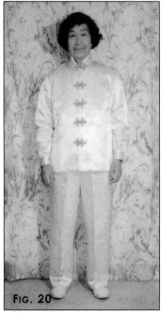

FIG. 20

Holy Wheel
Rotating Forever

This movement uses all the joints of the body: neck vertebra, chest vertebra, waist vertebra, shoulders, elbows, wrists, thighs, and ankles. All of these joints do a round cycle movement, left and right exchange. The posture can cure shoulder inflammations and rheumatism, as well as bringing the body into balance.

1. Stand naturally, feet parallel, shoulder width apart as shown in figure 21. Put the back of your left hand on the Mingmen

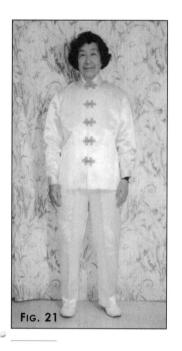

FIG. 21

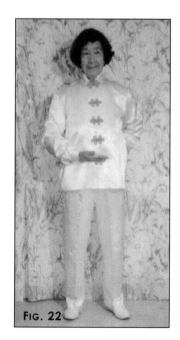

FIG. 22

acupuncture point (see glossary) on your back, opposite your navel. Put your right hand, palm upward, near the navel. Pay attention to relaxing the waist. See figure 22.

2. Inhale as you turn the upper part of your body to the left, toward the back as much as possible (figure 23). Following the body, slowly lift up your right hand in an arc from your navel to over your head. See figure 24.

3. As you turn your body to face front again, move your right hand up in front of your body, keeping your hand over your head, with your arm straight up, palm facing left. See figure 25 on page 30.

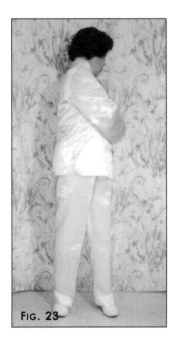

FIG. 23

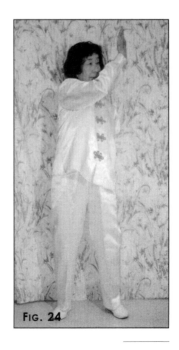

FIG. 24

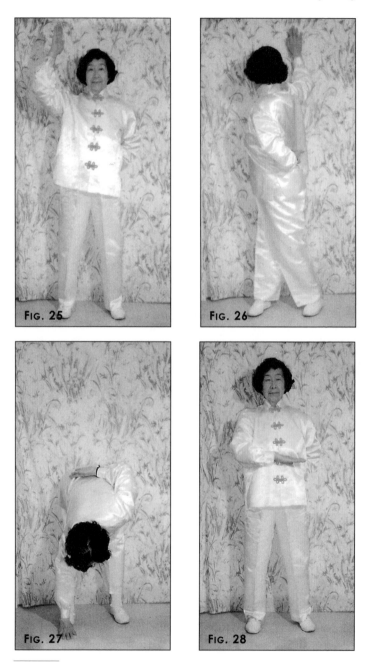

FIG. 25

FIG. 26

FIG. 27

FIG. 28

4. Bend down from your waist, bringing your right arm down until the palm of your hand touches the ground (as close to the ground as possible). Exhale. See figures 26 and 27.

5. Slowly stretching the waist, rotate the right palm up and raise it to Dan Tian, palm downward. Then turn up the palm over your head. See figures 28 and 29.

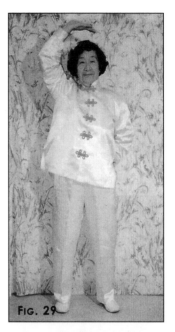

FIG. 29

6. Continue moving your right hand to the Mingmen point (see glossary) on your back and exchange places with your left hand. Consciously guide the Chi to slowly sink to the Dan Tian. The waist vertebra is like a holy wheel, rotating forever.

7. Continue the exercise with your left hand, palm upward,

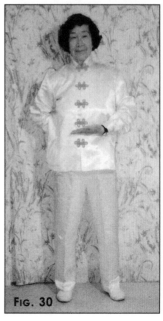

FIG. 30

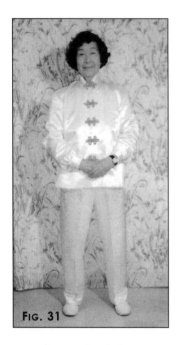

FIG. 31

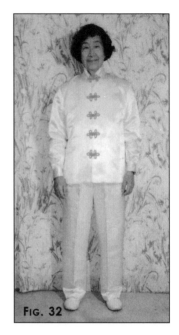

FIG. 32

near the navel, inhaling as you turn the upper part of your body to the right. The other movements are the same as in Step 6. Repeat these movements several times.

Squatting and Standing

STAND NATURALLY. With both hands stretching forward with palms upward (see figure 33 on page 34), fingers close together, raise your arms and palms as high as your shoulders, so that the Inside Laogongs of both hands receive (inhale) the Chi (vital energy) from the heavens. Inhale as you raise your hands. Exhale, as you slowly go down to a squatting position, as low as you comfortably can, keeping arms straight and palms upward (see figure 34). Come back to a standing position and do this again (see figures 35, 36). Always return to a standing position (figure 37).

When you inhale, your diaphragm is expanded and the abdominal wall protrudes. This is favorable breathing. In this way, you can inhale a lot of oxygen and fresh air. As you exhale, your diaphragm is contracted and the abdominal wall is concave. This kind of abdominal respiration should be an exercise that you perform to achieve greater movement in the diaphragm and abdominal wall.

The breathing movement is the key link in any breathing exercise. By training consciously, you can change your breathing

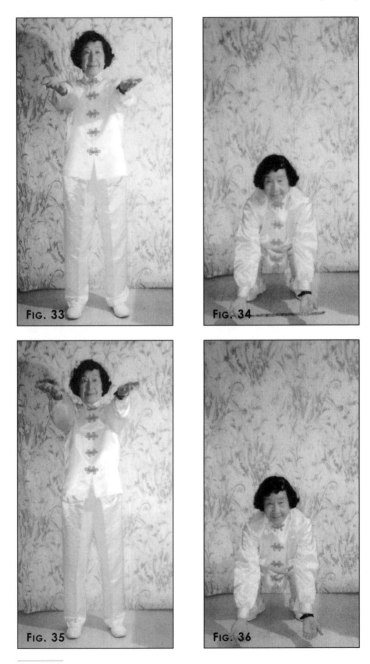

FIG. 33

FIG. 34

FIG. 35

FIG. 36

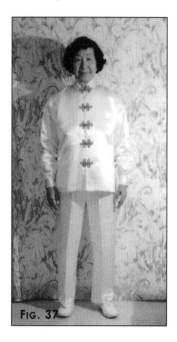

FIG. 37

from shallow to deep breathing. As a result of this, your vital capacity is increased, the gas metabolism and blood circulation are improved, digestion and absorption are improved. All these changes ensure the achievement of good health, the effectiveness of the treatment, disease prevention, and a strong body.

It is advisable to move slowly. Don't hurry. You should go step by step gradually and should not be overly anxious for quick results. You must remember the combination of practice and rest. Do not overwork the respiratory muscles. You should practice and cultivate your breathing to achieve a natural, smooth, and gentle breathing using these fundamental principles. After a few minutes of exercise, you should return to your normal breathing.

Walking Kung

WALKING KUNG is a Kung that is done in a walking position, but it is actually done standing in place. You do not need to be in a large area to do this exercise. It is nice to be outside, but you can also exercise inside. (When you practice inside, it is better to open the windows, in order to let the fresh air come in.) You can do this Kung anywhere, while you are at home, while you travel, on vacation, anywhere. It truly is a valuable practice.

This Kung is the basic Kung to prevent and cure diseases. Walking Kung is used for cultivating "true Chi," the Life Force of the human body. It is important that it is accompanied by breathing to provide a lot of oxygen to the internal organs so that it can increase nourishment, improve immunity, and regulate your metabolism. It is better to practice in the morning when the air is fresh. This Kung may be practiced anywhere as long as it is quiet and the Kung can be carried out without outside disturbance. The movements of the Walking Kung are simple, easy to learn, easy to practice, but the effect is great.

The starting posture for Walking Kung requires that you stand in an easy, relaxed position in a natural and comfortable state.

1. Empty your mind of all thought. Think about nothing. Drive away any kind of disturbances.

2. The feet should be shoulder width apart, with your toes pointing straight forward.

3. Start with both eyes looking ahead for a while, then slowly and gently close them lightly.

4. Your tongue should lightly touch the roof of your mouth, so that it can link up the Ren Channel with the Du Channel. This makes the nervous system of the teeth and mouth produce biological electricity.

5. The Baihui (crown of the head) should be up toward the sky. Imagine there is a thread from heaven pulling your Baihui upward.

6. Allow your shoulders to hand down and draw your elbows down. These three joints—wrists, elbows, and shoulders—must all be relaxed. If the shoulders are not relaxed, if both shoulders are up, the Chi will be lifted upward and will be unable to sink to the Dan Tian. The other joints must be relaxed for the same reason.

7. Don't hunch your back or bend your body backward. The chest should be held inward a little bit, so that the backbone will be erect. Hold your shoulders slightly, so as to empty the armpits and relax your wrists.

8. Relax the waist, and pull your abdomen inward.

9. With conscious thought, and no force, lift up the anus and Huiyin (perineum) slightly.

10. Rotate the tongue inside the mouth, and swallow the saliva three times. Imagine that you send the saliva down to the Dan Tian. Saliva can help your body's digestion and increase immunity to disease.

11. The mental and physical state of the body must be relaxed. It is especially important that the mind be relaxed and totally free of any thoughts; then the muscles of the whole body will be relaxed. All the joints of your body are relaxed as well. Your body gradually will become flexible, and will allow the Chi to flow fluently through every part of your body

Left Side Walking Kung

Stand naturally with your feet parallel, a shoulder width apart. Then move the weight of your body to the right leg and foot, slightly bending your right leg. Using the right foot as an axis, turn the body slowly to the left and forward. At the same time lift up the left leg and take one step forward, touching the heel of the left foot to the ground first, holding the toes upward. After the gravity of the body falls on the left foot, flatten the left foot.

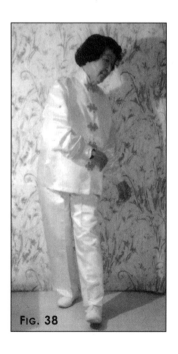

FIG. 38

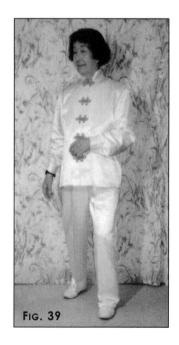

FIG. 39

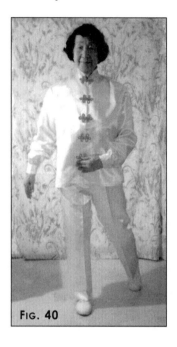

FIG. 40

The right hand slowly swings to the Dan Tian, but the hand does not actually touch the body. The left hand slightly swings to the outside downward region of the left thigh. When both hands are swinging, the waist, head, neck, and the body all follow in turning to the left. As the body bends slightly forward, gently pull in your abdomen. The whole body must be relaxed. The shoulders, elbows, and wrists should also be relaxed. Then return the left foot to its original place. Consciousness will also leave the Dan Tian. When you end this Kung, walk around slowly, and then take a rest.

Right Side Walking Kung

With the right foot, take a step forward. As the heel touches the ground the toes are up. The rest of the movements are the same as for Left Side Walking Kung.

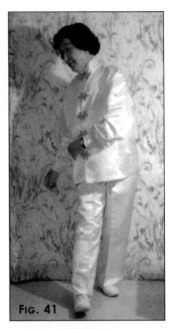

FIG. 41

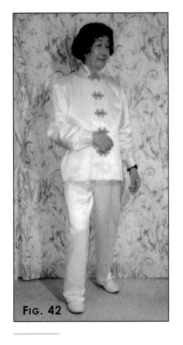

FIG. 42

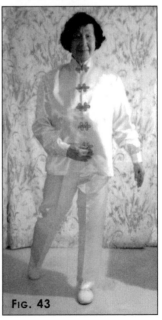

FIG. 43

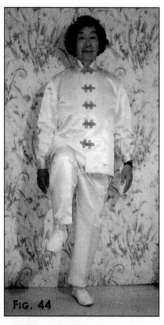

FIG. 44

Exchange Walking

Stand naturally. Bend your knees, and take 3 short steps walking first forward, then backward. This exercise improves muscle tone and stiffness and strengthens the back thigh muscles.

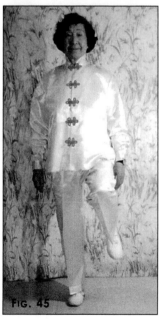

FIG. 45

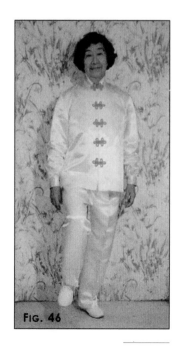

FIG. 46

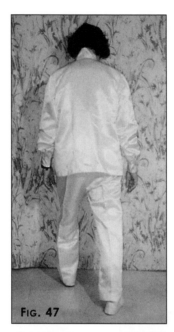

FIG. 47

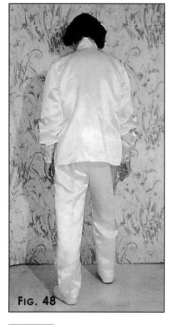

FIG. 48

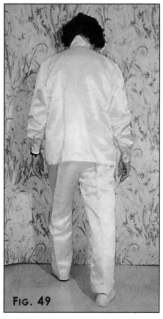

FIG. 49

Flat Three-Step
Walking Kung
(One-Two-Three, Three-Two-One)

Do free walking. Hands can be joined at your back or swing naturally at your sides. Take 3 steps forward; that is, left foot, right foot, 3 times. As you lift up your left foot and take your first step, inhale and hold through all three steps. Then exhale beginning with your right foot through the next three steps. The length of time between inhaling and exhaling is the same.

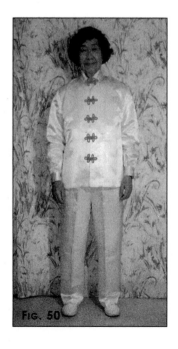

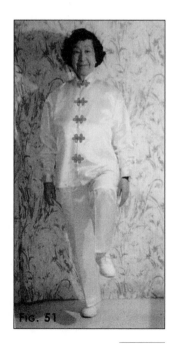

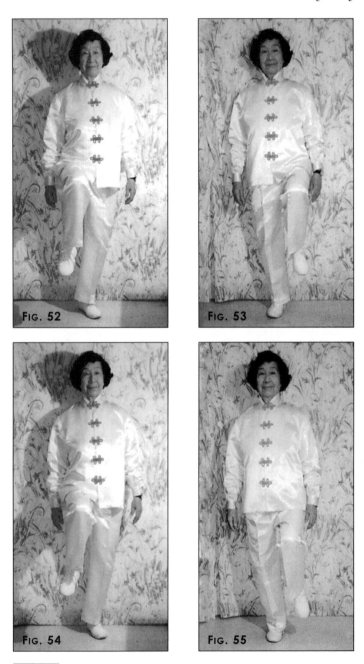

FIG. 52

FIG. 53

FIG. 54

FIG. 55

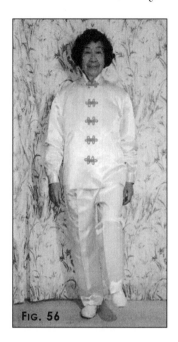

FIG. 56

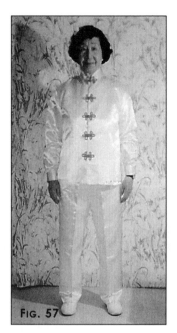

FIG. 57

There is no natural breathing done during inhaling and exhaling with this exercise. You should hold respiration (see page 12). When you inhale, you are breathing in the universal Chi. When you exhale, you are getting rid of the stale, negative Chi in your body.

Training Legs

IT IS VERY IMPORTANT to relax your knees. If the knees are not relaxed, the Chi (vital energy) cannot pass through to reach your feet. Some people, upon standing, feel a rush of Chi passing through the knees to the feet. Eventually, your feet will become warmer. This exercise strengthens the knees and feet.

1. Stand erect with your hands on either side of your waist with feet close together. Keep the torso erect. Relax your feet and knees.

2. Slowly bend your knees as shown in figure 58 on page 50. Hold your body slightly back (see figure 59) so that the thighs and torso make a straight line. Keep the head upward and slightly back. Lift your heels off the ground slightly.

3. Keep this posture as long as you comfortably can. Then stand up slowly. Repeat this movement three times.

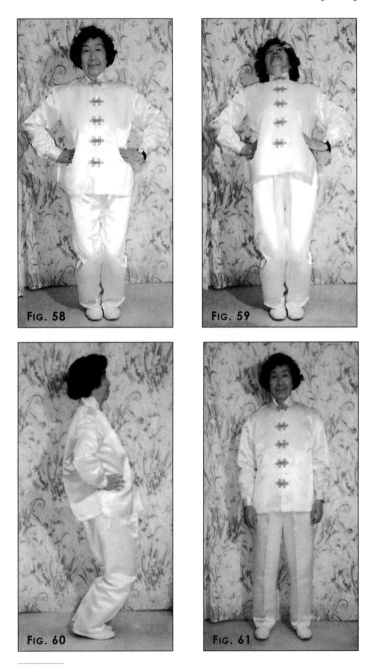

FIG. 58

FIG. 59

FIG. 60

FIG. 61

Lower Legs
and Feet

Tree begins to decay;
first of all, its roots rot.
A person begins to get old;
first of all, the feet
lose strength.

-ANCIENT CHINESE PROVERB

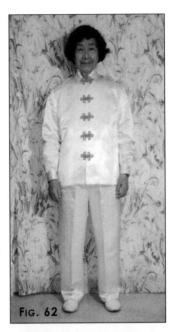

FIG. 62

If your feet are without energy, or lose strength, it is a sign that your body is beginning to get old. So you must train your legs and feet in order to increase strength and prevent spasms. To do this, use the following exercise.

1. Stand quietly with feet parallel (figure 62). Take a step forward with your left foot. The distance between both feet should be about two feet. Keep both feet flat on the ground (figure 63).

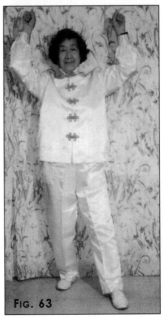

FIG. 63

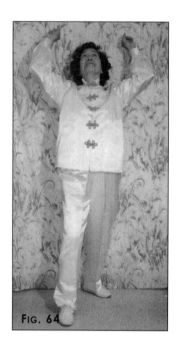

FIG. 64

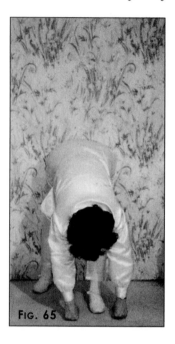

FIG. 65

2. Extend your hands and arms out to the sides, up and over your head, and very slowly bend down to the ground. Place your two fists on the ground on either side of your left foot. Your lower legs and thighs must be straight, and you should feel the muscles in the back of your legs and thighs stretching. Hold this posture for 30 seconds. See figures 64, 65.

3. Stand up very slowly. Don't hurry. Then change feet, and take a step forward with the right foot. Do this exercise again with the right foot forward. Figures 66 and 67 are back views of this exercise.

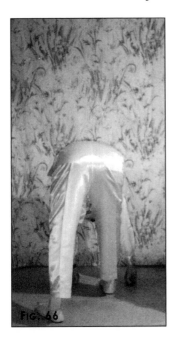

FIG. 66

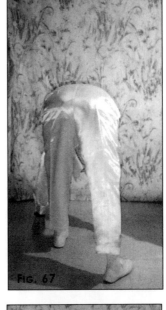

FIG. 67

Practice, alternating feet, several times. Later, you may increase the number of times. Never force yourself to practice. You should practice as long as you feel comfortable doing so.

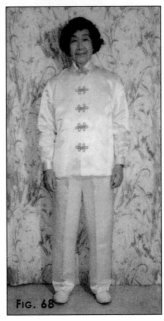

FIG. 68

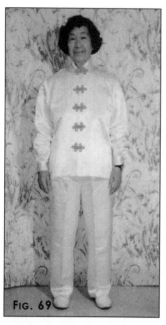

FIG. 69

Rotating Knees

1. Stand naturally with your arms and hands at your sides.

2. Squatting down, put your palms on your knees.

3. Rotate your knees from left to right in a circle (3 to 9 times).

4. Then rotate from right to left.

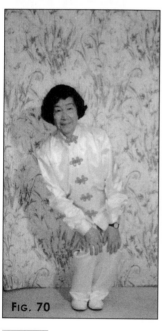

FIG. 70

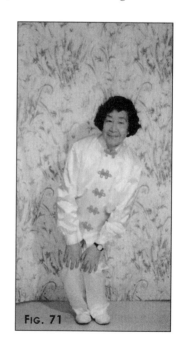

FIG. 71

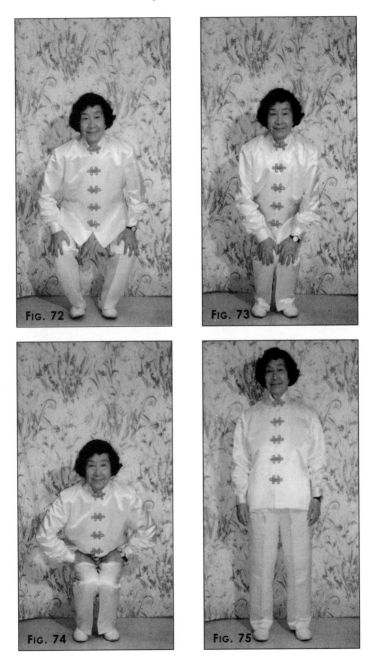

FIG. 72

FIG. 73

FIG. 74

FIG. 75

5. Then rotate from inward to outward, as shown figures 72 through 74 on page 55.

6. Rotate from outward to inward.

7. Then squat from a standing position, with your palms on thighs, fingers pointing inward, 3 to 9 times.

PART 2

Walking Kung

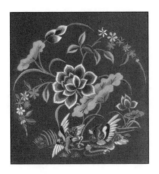

Chi Kung—Vital Energy for Life

It is the law of Nature
Which people have always believed;
That human beings made of earth
Are connected with the heavens.

One-Step Walking Kung

THIS KUNG IS beneficial for cultivating the life force of "True Chi" to strengthen the body's ability to prevent and fight diseases. It can greatly improve the function of immunity. It can also help in curing asthma.

1. Step forward with your left foot (figure 77). As the heel of your foot touches the ground, immediately breathe in two short "Inhale, Inhales." This is called Heel Inhaling. When the sole of your left foot is flat on the ground (figure 78), breathe out one short "Exhale." This is called Sole Exhaling.

2. Next, lift up your right foot and let the toes of your right foot lightly touch the ground (figure 79). This movement is called "Toes Dropping." Hold this "Toes Dropping" movement for a little while (figure 80). Then change to natural breathing. This posture is called "Taking Rest."

The whole process of One-Step Walking Kung includes four steps: (1) "Heel Inhaling," (2) "Sole Exhaling," (3) "Toes

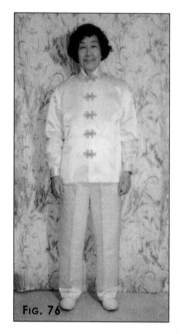

FIG. 76

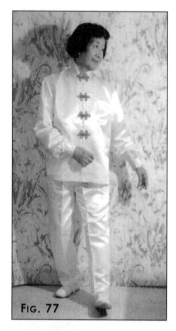

FIG. 77

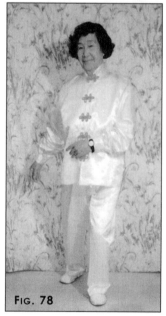

FIG. 78

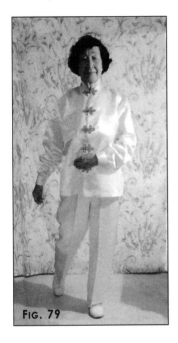

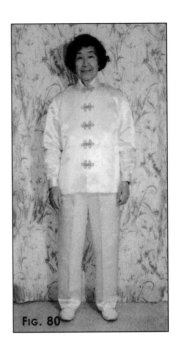

FIG. 79

FIG. 80

Dropping," and (4) "Taking Rest." Practice for a while. One-Step Walking Kung is also called Dropping Kung of Heel Inhaling and Sole Exhaling.

3. Now shift the weight of your body to your right leg and foot. Step forward with your left foot, and as the heel touches the ground, breathe two short "Inhale, Inhales." As you put the sole of your left foot on the ground, take one "Exhale." Then lift up your right foot as toes drop to the ground.

4. Then you "Take Rest" for one or two minutes with natural breathing. Then draw your right foot to the left, so both feet will be parallel. Practice for about twenty minutes. If you are weak

and cannot practice for twenty minutes each time, practice for five or ten minutes, or for as long as you feel comfortable. Gradually increase the time.

After twenty minutes of practice, you should rest by walking for fifteen to twenty minutes. In this way you can adjust your Chi.

Walking: Pay attention as you are walking. Look ahead and not at the ground. Don't let your hips protrude or hunch your back. Relax the whole body, the muscles and extremities, and above all, relax your mind.

Two-Step Walking Kung

THIS KUNG BENEFITS weak patients. It helps to inhale a lot of oxygen because fresh air can transform and produce internal Chi in your whole body.

1. Starting with the left foot, lift up your right hand to the Dan Tien. The left hand swings toward the left side of your left thigh. Meanwhile, the torso, head, and neck rotate slightly to the left side. The weight of the body falls on the right foot. Legs and knees are slightly bent, so that you are able to stand with stability. Slowly lift up your left foot and take a step forward. See figure 82 on page 64.

2. As the heel of your left foot touches the ground, toes pointing upward, breathe a short "Inhale." Following this movement, the weight of the body should fall on the right foot. After the left foot is flat on the ground, and the body is stable, lift up your right foot and take a second step as shown in figure 83 on page 64. Also as the heel of the right foot touches the ground, toes upward, breathe a short "Inhale" again. Following this movement, the weight of your body should fall on your left foot. After

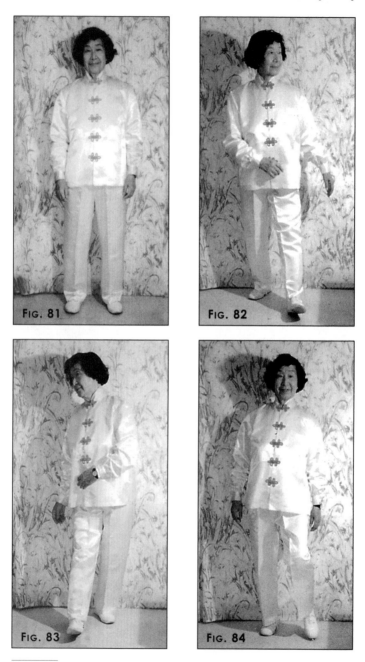

FIG. 81

FIG. 82

FIG. 83

FIG. 84

the right foot is put flat on the ground, and the body is stable, lift up your left foot and let the toes touch the ground and "Exhale" once. See figure 84.

3. Step forward two steps. On each step, as the heel touches the ground, make the sound of inhaling.

- First step: Slowly lift up your left foot and take one step forward. Let the heel touch the ground, toes pointing upward. Breathe a short "Inhale."

- Second step: Lift up your right foot and step forward. Let the heel touch the ground and breathe a short "Inhale" again.

4. After your right foot is flat on the ground, lift up your left foot, let the toes touch the ground and "Exhale." Now it is unnecessary for you to step forward one step again. You have already taken two steps. Then bring the back foot to the front, letting both feet be parallel, and do natural breathing. Practice for fifteen to twenty minutes. You may rest by walking fifteen minutes for the purpose of adjusting your Chi.

5. Continue to step forward one step with your left foot. As the heel touches the ground, breathe a short "Inhale." Then lift up your right foot, and as the heel drops down on the ground, breathe a short "Inhale." After your right foot is flat on the

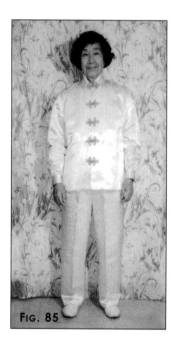

Fig. 85

ground, lift up your left foot. Let the toes drop to the ground and "Exhale." Then do natural breathing.

Remember, on each foot you can only step one step. Each time you step two steps with two feet, accompanied by breathing two short "Inhale, Inhales," and one "Exhale." End with natural breathing.

Three-Step Walking Kung

 THIS KUNG IS THE BEST way to improve the total level of health, and strengthen the internal Chi movement. It helps to lower blood pressure, and heal any inflammation of the liver. Do not walk or breathe too fast.

The special point of this Kung is that "Two Inhales, One Exhale" will be changed to use three steps. The quantity of breathing and the moving condition of internal Chi will be slow.

1. Start with the left foot. Move the left arm and hand to the left side of the thigh. Rotate the torso, head, and neck to the left, and bring the right arm and hand to the left, in front of the Dan Tian, as in figure 87 on page 68. The gravity of the body moves to the right leg and foot.

2. Lift up the left foot slightly and take one step forward. Heel touches the ground with toes up. At this time, breathe one short "Inhale." Then slowly put the left foot flat on the ground.

3. Move the right hand in front of the Dan Tian to the right side of the thigh. Move the left hand back to the front of the Dan Tian. The gravity of the body moves to the left leg and foot.

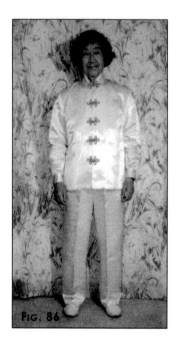
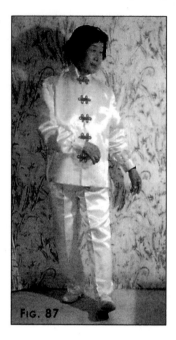

FIG. 86   FIG. 87

4. Rotate the torso, head, and neck. Turn your face slightly toward the right, as in figure 88.

5. Then lift up your right foot and take a step forward, heel touching the ground and toes up. Again breathe one "Inhale." Then put the right foot flat on the ground.

6. Move both hands toward the left side, the gravity of the body moving to the right foot. Turn the body forward toward the left. Lift up the left foot and take a step forward, touching the heel to the ground, toes up. At this time, "Exhale."

The first three steps you take should be accompanied by 2 "Inhales" and 1 "Exhale."

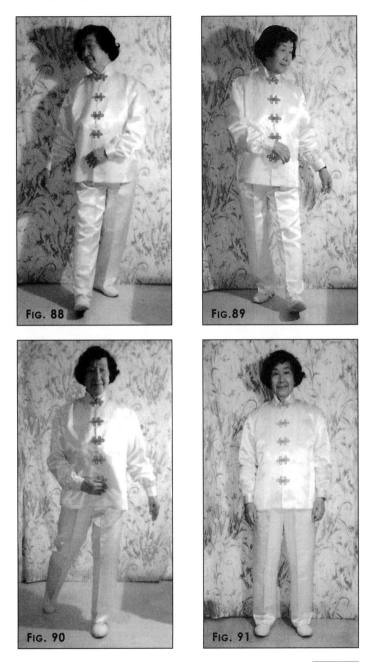

FIG. 88

FIG.89

FIG. 90

FIG. 91

After you finish taking these three steps, again put the left foot flat on the ground. Both arms and hands sway toward the right side. Move the weight of the body to the left leg and foot. At this movement, the right foot must not step forward again, and the toes are slightly touching the ground.

Relax the wrists and the joints of the arms and hands. Both hands should hang naturally by the sides of the body. Do "Forget Breathing"—natural breathing. This is also called "Pin Chi," letting the Chi slowly sink to the Dan Tian to increase vital energy and increase your life force.

Quick Walking Kung

THE IMPORTANT FUNCTION in this Kung is to dredge through the Kidney (Water), adjust the Spleen (Earth), benefit the Lung (Metal), nourish the Liver (Wood), and calm or quiet the Heart (Fire).

As in walking, pay more attention to the heel than to the sole of the foot. Although the name is Quick Walking, in fact, it is not very quick, just a "little quick." During practice, keep a relaxed and soft posture. Don't be stiff, and don't be in a hurry!

Right "Inhale," left "Exhale" is Yin Ascending, Yang Descending. Left "Inhale," right "Exhale" is Yang Ascending, Yin Descending.

1. Move your right hand from the right thigh to the front of your abdomen. Swing your left arm and hand toward the left outside of the thigh. The weight of the body moves to the right foot.

2. Lightly lift up your left foot and take one step forward. As the heel touches the ground, toes upward, breathe two short "Inhale, Inhales." After the left foot is flat on the ground, the weight of the body moves to your left foot.

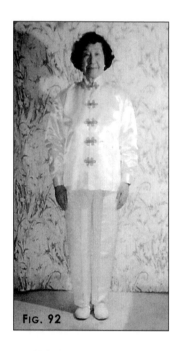

FIG. 92

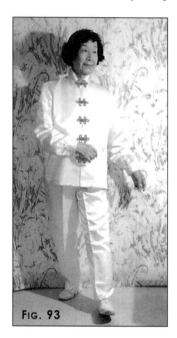

FIG. 93

3. Slightly lift up your right foot and take one step forward. As the heel touches the ground, toes upward, do one "Exhale."

4. Lift up your left foot and take a step forward. As the heel touches the ground, toes upward, breathe two short "Inhale, Inhales." After the left foot is flat on the ground, step forward with your right foot. As the heel touches the ground, toes up, do one short "Exhale."

5. Again, when the left heel touches the ground, breathe two short "Inhale, Inhales." As the right heel touches the ground do one "Exhale." Both feet change to step forward: left, right, left, right. When you have practiced about twenty minutes, bring

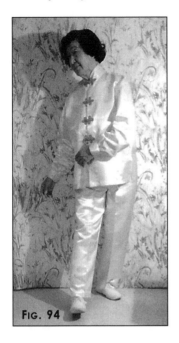

FIG. 94

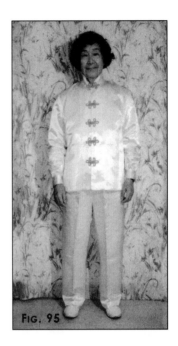

FIG. 95

your left foot to the front to be parallel with the right foot. Then take a rest for twenty minutes and do natural breathing.

6. If a person is too weak to walk, he or she may sit down, relax, empty the mind, and breathe naturally for twenty minutes.

Practice the whole process three times. From beginning to end is considered to be once. Although the name of this Kung is called "Quick Walking Kung," don't practice too fast. Above all, practice should be gradual to improve your skill and vital energy.

Don't hurry! Never hurry!

Quicker Walking Kung

 THIS KUNG IS CALLED "Heel Inhale, Sole Exhale" Kung. This Kung can quickly arouse the internal Chi so that it will move fluently through almost every part of the body.

1. On one foot, the practitioner should finish a complete process with two short "Inhale, Inhales" at the heel of the foot, and one "Exhale" at the sole of the foot. The heel and the sole must work.

2. Following the last movement, move your left arm and hand from the left thigh to the front of your abdomen. Swing your right arm and hand down toward the right outside of the thigh. The weight of the body moves to the left foot.

3. Lightly lift up your right foot and take one step forward. As the heel touches the ground, immediately breathe two short "Inhale, Inhales." Then as the sole touches the ground, breathe out one short "Exhale."

4. Lift up your left foot and take one step forward. As the heel touches the ground breathe two short "Inhale, Inhales." As the

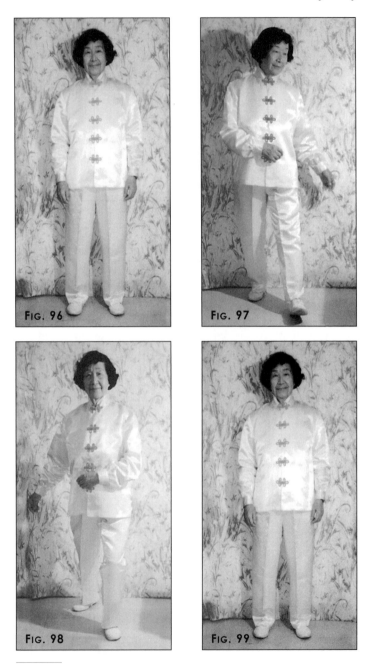

FIG. 96

FIG. 97

FIG. 98

FIG. 99

sole touches the ground, breathe out one "Exhale." Continue to step forward step by step.

Remember: on one foot, you must finish a complete process with two short inhales at the heel and one exhale at the sole. Don't forget the sole. The heel and sole must work. Both feet change and step forward, right, left, right, left.

At last, when you have practiced fifteen or twenty minutes, bring your left foot to the front parallel with your right foot. Take a rest for fifteen or twenty minutes. Then continue to practice three times.

Quickest Walking Kung

THIS KUNG IS THE strongest and is very fast. The special function of this Kung is to inhale a lot of oxygen. Most patients who suffer from chronic diseases have an oxygen deficiency. Practicing this Kung can save lives. Again, don't hurry! You need to practice a long time in order to cure chronic diseases thoroughly. The therapy of the Kung is to train yourself through Chi to be able to cure your diseases. It allows the whole body to heal the sickness, according to the patients' psychology and physiology. Chi is medicine. Chi can cure chronic diseases or prevent and fight cancer. Chi has wonderful, powerful, and miraculous effects.

1. Move your right hand from the right thigh to the front of your abdomen. Swing your left arm and hand toward the left side of the thigh. The weight of the body moves to the right foot.

2. Lightly lift up your left foot and take a step forward. As the heel touches the ground, immediately breathe one short "Inhale."

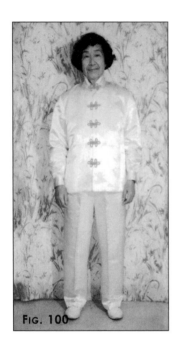
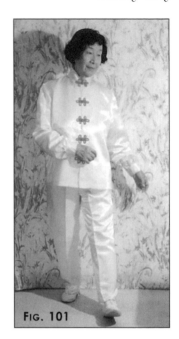

Fig. 100   Fig. 101

3. Lift up your right foot and take a step forward. As the heel touches the ground, toes upward, immediately breathe out one short "Exhale."

4. Practice five to ten minutes.

Remember: when you step forward with your left foot and your left heel touches the ground, breathe one "Inhale." Then when you step forward on your right foot and your right heel touches the ground, breathe out one "Exhale." It is: "One step, one Inhale, one step, one Exhale.

During your walk, your head, neck, shoulders, waist, thighs, hands, and eyes should be relaxed. Don't look down at the ground, look straight ahead.

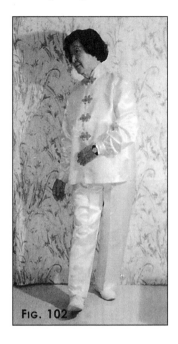

FIG. 102

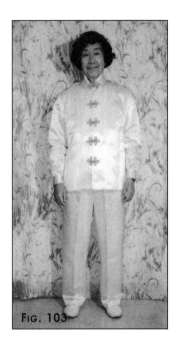

FIG. 103

When you finish the Kung, bring your back foot to the front and let both feet be parallel. Close both eyes slightly. Then slowly open your eyes.

This Quickest Walking Kung is the strongest. It uses "Heel Inhale and Heel Exhale." It is the best way to improve your kidneys and spleen, adjust your stomach and intestines, and also change negative emotions into good and delightful ones.

One should practice this Kung three times. After each time, take a rest. Then continue.

Ancient Chinese Traditional Five-Step Walking Kung

 IN ANCIENT TIMES, this Kung was called "Yin Links Up Yang," or "Yang Connects with Yin." Here "yin" refers to Earth, "yang" refers to Heaven.

First, the mind must be totally emptied of all thoughts, so that it completely thinks nothing. The whole body is emptied of all its strength. The overall process is to inhale more oxygen and to exhale less so that the body has an excess of oxygen. You should inhale and exhale through the nose. The tip of the tongue touches the roof of the mouth during this Kung. All kinds of chronic diseases will be driven away with this Kung. Many weak people, young and old, are suffering from chronic diseases, and cancer, and are oxygen deficient. Practicing this Kung is the best method for them.

It is recommended that for best results this Kung be practiced for two hours every morning. If you cannot practice it for two hours at a time, you may practice it for half an hour or even for 20 minutes. Then take a rest. Then continue to practice it some more. Gradually, you will be able to increase the length of time, as you become stronger and stronger. If you are too weak at first to practice longer, you may, in the beginning, practice as long as you feel comfortable. Never hurry!

This is a very important method which must combine practice with rest. That means you practice for a while, and then rest for a while so that the oxygen enters your body to improve your health. You will feel relaxed, peaceful, and comfortable.

To practice this Kung we use "rough breathing." When you inhale and exhale, you, yourself, can hear your breathing sound. You breathe with as much strength as comfortably possible so that you can hear the sound of your breath. Close your mouth and let the breathing sound come out of your nose.

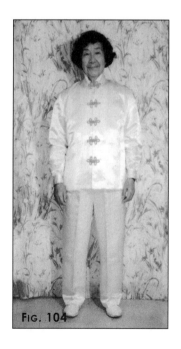

FIG. 104

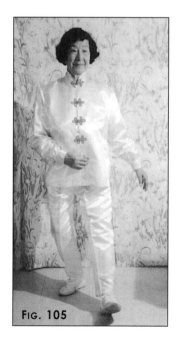

FIG. 105

1. With your weight on one foot, as the heel of the other foot touches the ground, inhale twice with your nose. While the sole touches the ground, exhale once with the nose with a "hu" sound. Regardless of which foot you use first, the method is the same.

2. After you step forward five steps (left, right, left, right, left), raise your right foot and let the toes touch the ground. At this moment, pronounce "sss"—this sound (Chi) comes out from between the tips of the teeth and the lips. Then put the sole of this foot flat on the ground in the same place. Take a 20-second rest, using natural breathing.

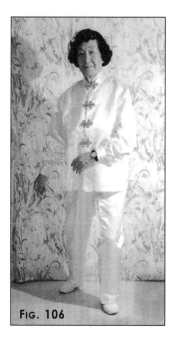

FIG. 106

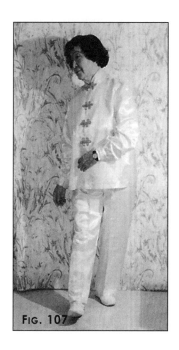

FIG. 107

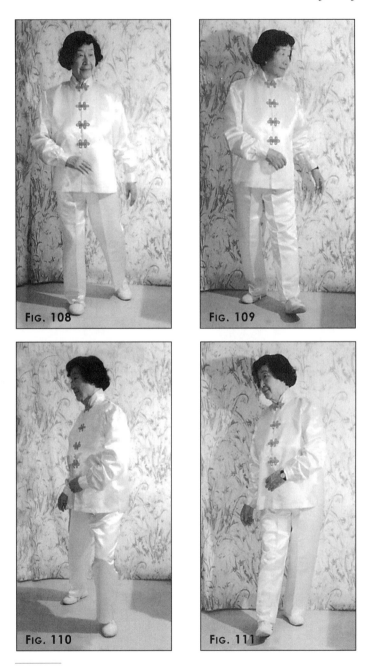

FIG. 108

FIG. 109

FIG. 110

FIG. 111

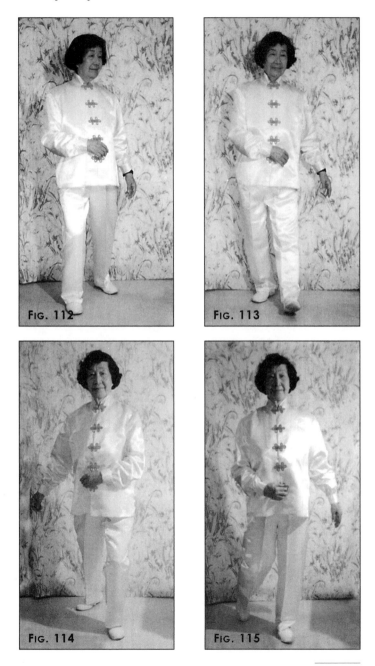

FIG. 112

FIG. 113

FIG. 114

FIG. 115

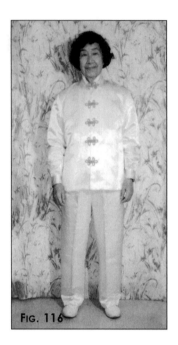

FIG. 116

3. Again, lift up your left foot, walk forward, and practice "shi, shi, hu" with the nose, then change to the right foot. As the heel touches the ground, do "shi shi" with the nose. As the sole is flat on the ground, do "hu." The method is the same as the above. Continue practicing as long as you feel comfortable.

4. As you are walking, you should relax your waist vertebra and sway arms and hands freely. Never use any energy.

Normal Reactions and Abnormal Reactions

IT IS NORMAL for most practitioners, after they have been practicing for a short or long time, to feel the internal Chi moving. They feel a slight electric feeling. Their hands become warm or numb. They experience this electricity on the armpits, waist, legs, and even the whole body. Sometimes it appears that the muscles are slightly jumping. During practice, they feel that their joints are squeaking. Some feel hungry and want to eat, some want to sleep. They also have high spirits. The whole body is relaxed, light, and comfortable.

Abnormal reactions are those that some people feel when their heels are painful after practicing Walking Kung. The way to correct this is, as you practice Walking Kung, to slightly touch your heels to the ground, but never use heavy weight. Never!

Some people feel a nose pain or a headache, or dizziness. To correct this, as you practice Walking Kung, inhale and exhale through your nose. Do not over exert your breathing function. If you use heavy breathing, it will produce abnormal reactions. When you breathe through your nose, the sound that you, yourself, can hear is enough. Never attempt to use strength! Don't practice too fast! Continue as long as you feel comfortable and cheerful. If you feel uncomfortable, you may adopt "Forget Breathing"—natural breathing—to adjust your breath. It helps the whole body relax.

The Miracle—
The Little Girl
and the Tortoise

IT WAS DURING the war and the man had carried his daughter on his back for five days. Their village was behind them in ruins, and the man could hear the firing of the guns in the distance as he tried to get away from the advancing enemy.

On the outskirts of an abandoned village, they sat down on a pile of stones and began to eat the last of their food. Tomorrow, starvation would be their new companion. How would he be able to forage for food and also look out for her? He looked at her tiny face and tears welled up in his eyes. Suddenly, he began to pull at the stones on which they were seated. In a minute he had uncovered an opening in the ground.

Carefully, he lowered himself, using the inner stone wall as a ladder. A narrow slit of light shown from above and revealed that the well was shallow and dry. Steeling himself, he went back for the girl. When he had placed her against a stone and wrapped her in her mother's jacket, he held her briefly and then climbed back up the wall and disappeared into the war zone. She would be one more uncounted victim, but the enemy troops would not find her.

◆ ◆ ◆

THE OLD MAN had the face of a jackal who has been running and hiding and existing on scraps all his life. He moved quickly through the village, as if he had on his mind a secret destination. When he reached the pile of stones, his heart soared and then sank again. He could see her bones already, and the memory of her innocent face filled him with remorse. He removed the last stone and descended into the darkness.

He scuffed his feet in the dirt and waited for his eyes to focus in the dark. All he could make out were a few loose rocks. Suddenly, there was a movement in the corner. He stiffened. Was there an animal living here? "Father," came the small voice, "Is it you?" So, her ghost was here to greet him, he thought. Again, a wave of shame and grief came over him, as he remembered his cruel decision to abandon her. He closed his eyes. There was a pressure on his arm. Her hand?

After they sat for a while, she told him her story. "During the first days the hunger was not so bad, but then I began to have pains here . . . in my chest. They grew worse, and I thought I was going to die. One day I was sitting against the wall, and I heard a small noise. I looked up and saw him in the corner. He was stretching his neck in and out of his shell in very slow movements. As I watched him, I started to imitate what he was doing. I stretched my neck out each time he did, and then I pulled it in.

In a few minutes I had forgotten my hunger and I felt nourished. I began to follow his movements all around the dark room where we lived. Another day, I saw him pull his head and neck into his shell like this." She showed her father the exercise she had learned from the tortoise. "In this way, learning to live like the tortoise, I passed my days and months until you came for me. I am only sad that we must now part."

Her father got up and began to look around for the tortoise. "No, he must stay. This is his home. It is enough that he has taught me to live on nothing, like a tortoise .... Can we go?"

The story of the little girl and the tortoise was published in magazines and newspapers all over China. The exercises she learned by closely observing the tortoise have been passed on to others. They are called "Turtle Kung." Those who use them experience the same life-enhancing energy that she felt as she imitated the tortoise in her dark room.

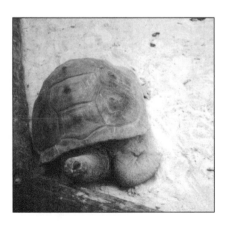

Glossary of Terms

Baihui. The point at the top of the head; the crown.

Changqiang. The point located on the coccyx or tail bone; the starting point of the Du Channel.

Chengjiang. Point in the middle of the depression between lower lip and chin.

Daimei. Belt Channel, waistline; begins under the navel, where it divides into two branches which extend around the waist to the small of the back.

Dan Tian. A point three fingers below the navel. This point can be called the "sea" for the Chi of the whole body.

Deimei. See *Daimei*.

Dumai. Du Channel—runs along the spinal column from the Changqiang, the neck, to the skull, over the crown of the head to the roof of the mouth. This channel is very strong, connecting the nervous system of the body. It passes through 28 acupuncture points located mostly along the spine.

Empty Fists. Fingers naturally close together with the thumb touching the tip of the middle (long) finger. Palms are empty.

Huiyin. Perineum; the point between the anus and the genital organ.

Joyu. The region of the kidneys.

Laogong. The point near the center of the palm (Inside Laogong); Outside Laogong is located in the center of the back of the hand. "Lao" equals "work, labor"; "Gong" equals palace. This point is very important in the treatment of diseases.

Mingmen. The point on the lower back, opposite the navel. This is a very important point through which the vital energy of life goes in and out; it is a gate.

Renmai. Ren Channel—goes through the center and front of the body. It begins at the perineum and extends up to the base of the mouth. When the tongue rests against the palate, it forms a bridge between dumai and renmai. This channel has 24 acupuncture points.

Shengyu. These two points are located on both sides of the mingmen. They store up water for the proper functioning of the kidneys.

Tianmu. A point between the eyebrows, just below the center of the forehead; also referred to as the "Third Eye." It is the point of clarity.

Yingtan. The point located above and between the eyebrows. This is where Chi enters the head to benefit the brain.

APPENDIX 1

Acupuncture Points and Energy Channels

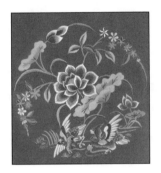

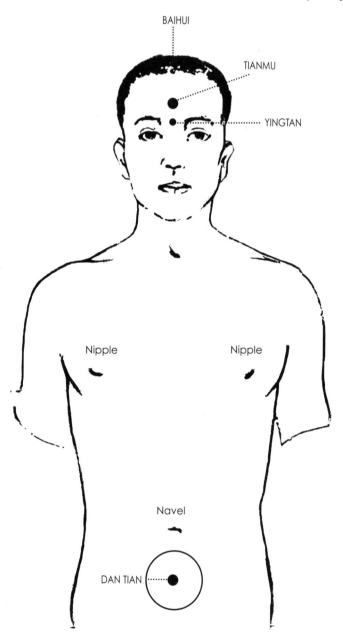

Dan Tian and the Major Acupuncture Points

In descending order from the top of the skull:

Baihui: At the top of the head; crown.

Tianmu: Between the eyebrows, just below the center of the forehead. The "Third Eye."

Yingtan: Between the eyebrows.

Dan Tian: The point three fingers width below the navel.

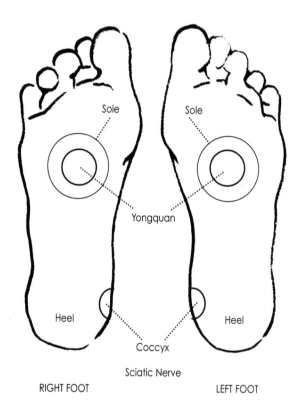

The feet, the roots of the body. Feet are the reflexes of the body's organs, glands, and limbs.

1

Bai *(hundred, all)*, **Hui** *(meet)*
This point is at the top of
the head.

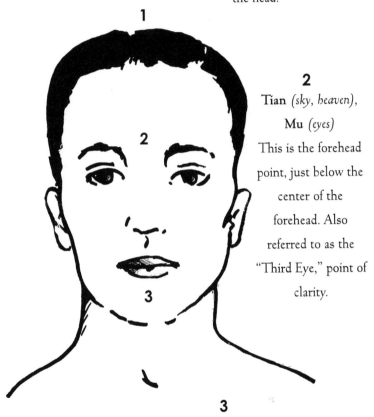

2

Tian *(sky, heaven)*,
Mu *(eyes)*
This is the forehead
point, just below the
center of the
forehead. Also
referred to as the
"Third Eye," point of
clarity.

3

Cheng *(receive)*, **Jiang** *(saliva)*
This point is in the middle of the
depression between the lower lip and
the chin. Saliva collects at this point.

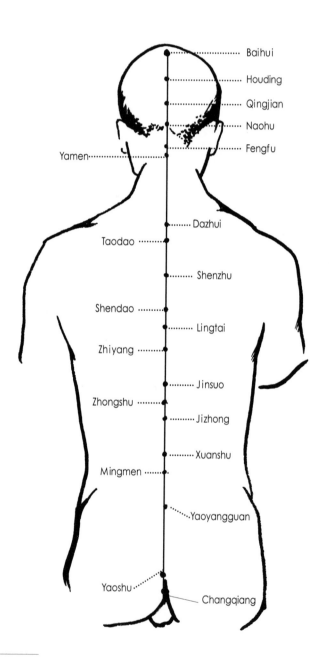

Baihui

Houding

Qingjian

Naohu

Fengfu

Yamen

Dazhui

Taodao

Shenzhu

Shendao

Lingtai

Zhiyang

Jinsuo

Zhongshu

Jizhong

Xuanshu

Mingmen

Yaoyangguan

Yaoshu

Changqiang

Du Mai (Du Channel)

Du *(govern)*, **Mai** *(vein)*

This is a channel that begins at Changqiang. This channel is very strong, connecting the nervous system of the body. It passes through 28 acupuncture points located mostly along the spine. At the nape of the neck (or back), this channel enters the brain, moving through Baihui, around on the forehead and ending at a point at the front of the hard palate (roof of the mouth).

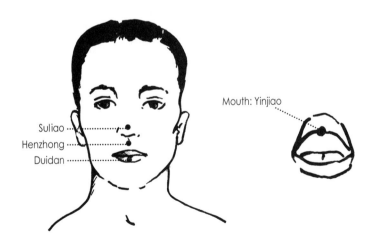

Mouth: Yinjiao

Suliao

Henzhong

Duidan

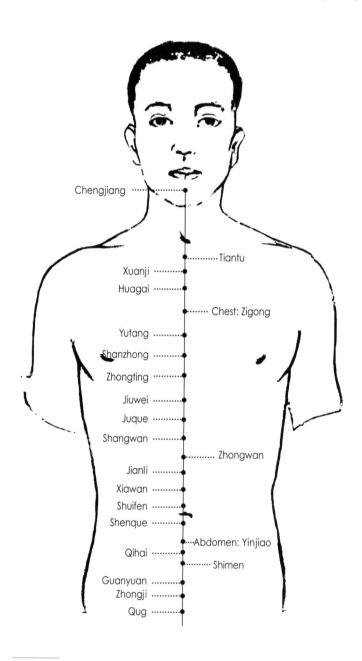

Chengjiang

Tiantu
Xuanji
Huagai
Chest: Zigong
Yutang
Shanzhong
Zhongting
Jiuwei
Juque
Shangwan
Zhongwan
Jianli
Xiawan
Shuifen
Shenque
Abdomen: Yinjiao
Qihai
Shimen
Guanyuan
Zhongji
Qug

Ren Mai (Ren Channel)

Ren *(appoint)*, **Mai** *(vein)*

The Ren Channel arises from the lower abdomen and emerges from the perineum. It ascends along the interior of the abdomen, and the front midline to the throat, up to the Chengjiang. The Ren Channel has 24 points.

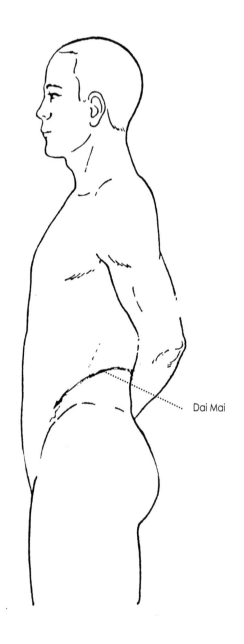

Dai Mai

Dai Mai

Dai *(belt)*, **Mai** *(meridian, vein)*

This is the line or meridian that circles the waist. "Holy Wheel Rotating Forever" dredges into the channel of Dai Mai.

Huiyin

Hui *(meet, converge)*, **Yin** *(meridian, perineum)*

This point is at the lowest part of the abdomen. It is a place where Yin energy gathers and three meridians—the Ren Channel, Du Channel, and Chong (Vital) Channel—meet together. It is a very important point. It is in the center of the perineum, between the anus and the scrotum in males and between the anus and the posterior labial commissure in females.

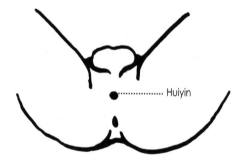

Yong Quan

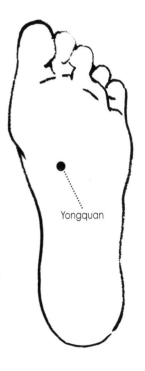

Yongquan

Yong *(gush out, well up),*
Quan *(spring, fountain)*

This acupuncture point is on the sole of the foot. The meridian energy moves up into the body from this acupuncture point, just as water springs from a fountain. This acupuncture point is very important, and it is considered as a second heart in Traditional Chinese Medicine.

APPENDIX 2

Testimonials

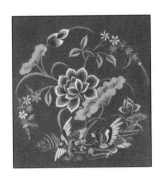

OCTOBER 6, 1993

Today was wonderful. We practiced and learned one "Ancient Chinese Walking Kung to increase life force and immunity to disease."

The energy moved through my body and I felt very peaceful. It is a way to focus inward and begin to understand how Chi can increase in your body. You can actually begin to feel it move. This is a very powerful Kung.

Thank you,

Patricia Robinson

AUGUST 27, 1995

We practiced today an exciting Kung which focuses on eliminating disease and prolonging life. As I continue to practice these amazing Kungs I feel my body becoming stronger and my mind becoming more peaceful. These are two of my long term goals—and the Chi Kung is such a powerful way to achieve this.

I'm realizing more and more that this practice slowly increases my ability to discover my inner resources—especially in times of stress. This is an awareness I didn't have before. My life is becoming richer after each experience I have with my practice.

Since I lead a very stressful life, the changes I have made internally through these exercises are invaluable.

Thank you, as always, for a wonderful session.

Patricia Robinson

JULY 19, 1993

Prevent Cancer Kung

I just recently arrived from a long trip—by plane and by car. I felt a little disoriented, tired, generally out-of-sorts. I began this cancer Kung with Professor Sheng this morning, and I feel so revived and have increased my energy a lot. I feel my head is much clearer, and certainly after 40 minutes my mental and physical energy and well-being has changed a good deal. I can notice immediately the effects which are all positive, from this Kung.

Julia Morin-Wisner

NOVEMBER 1, 1993

Prevent and Cure Cancer Kung

It must be directly related to the breathing done during this Kung that makes me so incredibly relaxed internally—both mentally and physically.

My stomach ceases grumbling and I can feel my digestive juices begin to flow quickly. Usually my mouth is very dry, but with this Kung, I have no dryness. Usually I have tightness in my shoulders, but practicing this Kung lubricates my joints.

I certainly feel more energy and feel more internally rejuvenated with this Kung.

Julia Morin-Wisner

APRIL 10, 1995

Monday

Today I came to practice Chi Kung, "Prevent Cancer Kung," with Professor Sheng. I felt very tired and not a lot of energy.

During the practice, I could feel sensations of hot energy up and down my body. I began to feel very peaceful and began to really enjoy it.

When I finish my practice, I feel more tranquil and full of mental energy. I feel very good.

Julia Morin-Wisner

Appendix 2

Recently I have learned four parts of Chi Kung: Vital Energy for Life to Increase Life Force and Improve Immunity to Disease. The first three parts work directly with breathing and moving the Chi through the body. Three Chi Breathing is very relaxing and allows my mind to become quiet and focused. I feel very calm and natural.

While practicing Three Opening and Closing, I can feel the Chi flowing between my hands and also centering around the Dan Tian. Although it is a quiet and conscious movement, it arouses a powerful feeling of the Chi in the center of my body. During Ascending and Descending Opening and Closing, I am very conscious of moving the Chi inside my body while gathering the Chi outside my body through the Inside and Outside Laogong. This is a very energizing movement. At the same time I feel totally relaxed and in control of the energy. The fourth part, Walking Kung, is very unusual and, although simple, is very difficult to coordinate at first. The sole-toe stepping, while breathing, turning the waist ever so slightly, moving hands and arms, and also turning the head simultaneously is challenging and requires concentration. After practicing a while, my waist and chest felt relaxed and the movements became effortless. The breathing technique is energizing and also cleared up my allergy symptoms!

Since I first learned Tai Chi from Professor Sheng many years ago, I have become very aware of the Chi that is everywhere and have learned how to direct it through the parts of my body that need healing. Thank you, Professor Sheng, for guiding me to this knowledge.

Judith Faria

Appendix 2

MAY 11, 1996

*Over the past ten years, I have had the unique opportunity
of knowing Professor Sheng and learning, not only many beneficial
exercises, but also a new way of looking at the world and my
place in it. The first and most difficult set I learned from her was
Ru Yu Tai Chi Chuan. Its complex and intricate movements (168
of them!) intrigue me, and I was determined to learn this fluid,
dance-like form. With my perseverance and Professor Sheng's
patience, I succeeded. I also learned Flying Crane Kung, Dragon
Swimming Kung, and Mu Lan Chuan.*

*Recently I have begun studying some exercises which in
China are practiced to cure and prevent cancer. It helps to
strengthen the immune system. The exercises focus on breathing and
walking, legs and feet training. After practicing, I feel refreshed,
energized, and healthier because of the respiration techniques.*

*All the forms I have learned have made me very aware of
the Chi inside me and in the universe, and of how to direct the
Chi in my body for self-healing . . . a great gift. It has been a
wonderful discovery, and I can now understand Professor Sheng's
life-long devotion to Chi Kung and its benefits.*

Judith Faria

AUGUST 17, 1993

I arrived late to class today, was very anxious and tense. We practiced Walking Kung and Silent Counting Kung. Almost immediately my mind became quieter and my body relaxed. While practicing I thought of nothing and felt the rhythm of the movements. When I finished my whole body felt relaxed but awake, my mind was clear and calm, my vision clear and I felt very happy and peaceful.

After the final movement, my hands were hot, my spine and neck were relaxed and I could feel the Chi in my back. To begin with my neck was stiff but after a moment's practice, my neck became loose and the exercise was easy. A wonderful alternative to Alexander Technique; much quicker.

This is two days in a row now. Yesterday I was stressed and bit by bit practicing Walking Kung, my mind became calm and happy and my body relaxed, full of energy, and color returned to my face.

Christina Corkill

AUGUST 21, 1993

I first met Professor Sheng three years ago. I had been studying Tai Chi but knew it was not what I wanted to learn. The answer came with meeting her and Chi Kung. While Tai Chi I found introspective, Chi Kung helped me get in touch with universal energy. My work often exhausted me but by practicing Chi Kung my energy and ability increased. Chi Kung restores the balance, reduces stress, and helps the body stay relaxed.

Returning to England I could find no one to teach me to the same level as Professor Sheng. Her understanding of Chi Kung is the result of learning under both Buddhist and Taoist masters, and many years of research.

Before leaving China, Professor Sheng prepared over thirty sets of Chi Kung and Tai Chi Chuan, some involving more than one hundred movements. She is still researching into the medical application of Chi Kung. It is this which brought me back to America and I have spent the last two months studying Chi Kung and its effects on stress-related illness, in the hope that I may be able to teach others on my return to England.

Christina Corkill

AUGUST 31, 1993

Today was my last Chi Kung lesson before I return to England. We learned Loose Waist Kung. This is a very relaxing Kung. It helps the joints to move more easily. It is important to practice slowly so that the waist and movements are relaxed. After we reviewed Shen Yun Kung. I could clearly feel the Chi as I practiced. Always as I practice now I am aware of the Chi and how my body feels. When I practice Chi Kung my mind and body are always relaxed. Sometimes it is difficult to "think of nothing" as Professor Sheng instructs, but even this seems possible at times. I have learned a great deal of Chi Kung, and although at the end of a class I may feel tired, afterward I have much more energy. I thank Professor Sheng for all her help, instruction, and kindness.

Christina Corkill

Appendix 2

MARCH 18, 1996

The movement today, "Walking Kung for increased life force and improving immunity," is very powerful. I felt my Chi in the Dan Tian gradually rise, like mist over a warm lake of water. I felt very mellow and energized throughout my whole body. Also, the weight of the body becomes lighter, with more flexibility in movement. The breathing is much deeper—not shallow like before the movement. The body is much more alive and flowing as a running water stream.

Thank you, Professor Sheng, for the remarkable, powerful energy that is stimulated within the body—it strengthens the body in total wholeness and well-being.

Robert Lew

OCTOBER 11, 1993

During practicing the Kung, especially the ascending, opening-closing one, I could feel the Chi moving through my tight shoulders when I had my hand above my head. It was pulling in my armpit and on the way down (when I lowered my hands) I could feel the warmth of the Chi flowing from my shoulders down my arm, into my hands.

While practicing the descending opening-closing Kung, I had similar feelings in my hips.

Monika Timpel

Appendix 2

Practicing the Kung of Relaxation and Tranquillity
Ascending and Descending, opening and closing, made me sweat.
The Chi moved to my feet and fingers. I could feel the Chi moving
out of my tight places: legs and shoulders. It is still difficult to
relax my shoulders but I let them drop more on the ascending
opening part.

My saliva production increased. I felt very relaxed and
peaceful after practicing.

Thank you.

Monika Timpel

JULY 12, 1992

Today I practiced Cancer Kung. I very much felt it in my hands at first. When the Laogong points crossed and I had my hands on my Dan Tian, I felt tremendous heat in them. I could feel the heat enter my body at the Dan Tian. I began to relax deeply in my body and my mind. When I separated my hands, opening and closing, I could still feel the heat and much energy, which also spread into my arms. Then when I began the ascending movement, I felt my body open up, especially the chest area. When I practiced the descending movement, I felt a very relaxed feeling in my whole body. I have more energy now than when I came today.

Jane Golden

Appendix 2

Today I continued to practice and learn Cancer Kung. When I came I felt tired. In the middle of practice I wanted to go to sleep. Now I feel very good. I feel very calm and relaxed. The first part is wonderful. I can feel and "see" the Chi in my whole body. I can feel opening and closing in my whole body. The second part I can move the Chi with my hand and consciousness. I can feel my whole body relax and I can feel hot and cold sensations in my arms. When I come down in front and bend forward to relax my waist, I can feel warmth in my legs. I can feel my shoulders relax deeply around the shoulder blade, and I can feel the blood go into my head.

I also learned part 3, but I could not yet relax enough to "feel" the result of it. Professor Sheng has also told me very much about this Kung Breathing, etc. I enjoy the information very much. It increases my understanding and makes a more complete experience.

Jane Golden

JUNE 7, 1986

Through the sessions of Chi Kung, I have noticed an increase of energy that allows me to go through an entire day of working and leave work energized rather than fatigued. I find myself able to draw on energy resources I didn't know I had.

I have also noticed a growing rejection of heavy and junk food by my body which is now signaling its wishes to be lighter and more energetic.

I am also beginning to sense Chi as a form of universal energy which enters my body, then flows back out again to the universe. This has led to an increasing feeling of being at one with nature and nature's consciousness. I love the feeling of being at home in the wind, the sunshine, the clouds and rain, receiving and giving back the energy of all life.

Thank you for furthering my quest for this understanding.
Gina Vaughn

Appendix 2

The measure of the cancer activity in my body, called PSA (Prostate Specific Antigen), has decreased since I started taking your class in Chi Kung.

I get a checkup at the National Institutes of Health in Bethesda, Maryland, every three months.

Will Collins

NOTE: *He had several checkups at the National Institutes of Health and every time he went, he found the cancer had decreased.* —AUTHOR

JULY 15, 1993

Today I arrived at Professor Sheng's with a terrible headache at the top of my Baiwei. So much so that I couldn't recall the first movements of Cancer Kung. After 2 sets of the opening, my headache began to go away. Within 40 minutes it was gone.

I feel better now, and feel more energy.

Frankie Eates

Index

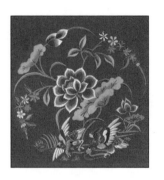

Index

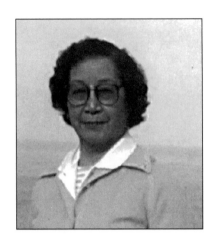

SHENG KENG YUN learned Chi Kung when she was very ill. Her health improved so dramatically that she became completely involved in working with Chi Energy. She has spent nearly forty years researching, mastering, and teaching Taoist, Buddhist, and Medical Chi Kung, as well as Tai Chi Chuan. A native of Kunming, China, she has degrees from three universties: Yunnan University, the Harbin Foreign Language Institute, and San Francisco State University. She has taught English and Russian at Yunnan University, is a member of the prestigious Chinese Chi Kung Scientific Academy, and author of *Key to Spoken English*. She lives in San Francisco, where she has been teaching people with special conditions for over ten years. She welcomes contact with students, and anyone wishing to contact her can do so by writing to Samuel Weiser, Box 612, York Beach, ME 03910.